Learn Spanish with Music
For Nurses

6-Step Formula to Remember Vocabulary

By: Inger Stapleton

Copyright © 2020 by Inger Stapleton

Part One: Debieras y Puedes

I. Why Nurses Should Learn Spanish   9
- About the book
- Learning Spanish vs. Speaking Spanish

II. Language Short Circuit   21
- Use Your Phone
- Crutches
- Second Language Superpower
- The Best Part

III. My Story   33
- Learning Journey
- Street Cred
  - Volunteering
  - A Different Perspective

IV. A Case for Music   45

Part Two: Imposible

V. Lies We Believe   51
- Kids Can, Adults Can't
- No Good at Languages

VI. Inspiration Lost   57
- No Time
- Constant Starter
- Lack of Comprehension
- No Progress

- Mistakes
- Context
- Why
- Excuses Be Gone

Part Three: Música

VII. Solution Overview   69
- Learn with Music
  - Learning Lifestyle
  - No Extra Time Needed
- The Basics
- Benefits of Music
  - Life Inspired Lessons
  - Native Context
  - Learn and Remember
  - Fun Education

VIII. Formula Breakdown   83
- Vocab as Building Blocks to Convos
  - Vocabulary = Communication
  - Es Como = It's like
- Step One: Artists, Songs & Genres
- Step Two: Lyrics
  - Accent Challenge
- Step Three: Accuracy
- Step Four: Translate

- Step Five: Mimic
- Step Six: Remember

Part Four: Mas que Palabras
IX. The *Doing* Challenge   97
- Use It; Don't Lose It
- Correction: Study Buddy
- Practice Groups
- More than Words

Appendix:
Starter Spanish Playlist – 101
Pre-made songs available on YouTube
search for "VocabBlocks"

» Part One «

Chapter One:
Capítulo Uno
Why Nurses Should Learn Spanish

During the Coronavirus pandemic millions of people stop in their tracks at 7:00 pm sharp daily to applaud nurses in unison from their front doorsteps. We say thank you for their sacrifice and care. We want them to hear us as they walk through their hospital halls and switch shifts.

Daily news outlets and YouTube videos have helped us understand the plights and fights of nurses for our lives on a whole new level. Before the pandemic, visiting a hospital when you're sick already had twilight zone characteristics. I was hospitalized for the first time in my life after the birth of my son in December of 2016.

When I went to the Emergency Room, I was told that the doctors needed to monitor my condition. The recent birth combined with my health issue was a cause for alarm, but they weren't sure what was wrong with me. The stress of not going home to my 6-day old baby was intoxicating but not knowing what was wrong with me was even more fear inducing.

Fortunately, on my first night in the hospital I had a caring nurse who did everything in her power to comfort and calm me. She shared personal stories with me about being a mom herself. She had an infant at home and a toddler. Within a few trips to my room she made me feel like she was a family member instead of a sterile caretaker, it had a tremendous positive impact on the most incredibly difficult experience of my life.

I was in excruciating pain and had a high fever. My nurse, Raquel, spoke to me calmly while asking my husband if he wanted to stay the night at the hospital and sleep next to me. She asked if we were hungry and offered food and drinks. When the food came, I couldn't eat but the gesture was reassuring. Her tone of voice felt like peace itself. It gave me the confidence that she had my best intentions at heart and would take good care of me.

I was trying to wrap my mind around the reality of what was happening; *'I'm sick, I can't go home, but I need to get to my baby. My baby needs me, will my baby know I'm his mom.'* While also trying to figure out what was going on with my body. My attempt to process what was going on meant I needed to ask more questions, but I didn't want to be a pest.

I was in a temporary holding location where doctors wanted to monitor my symptoms before admitting me officially into the hospital. I was hoping that they would send me home soon so I could be with my baby again. Unfortunately, my temperature remained high and my pain was steadily increasing.

When asked about my history, the medicine I had taken and if I had eaten before coming to the hospital, Raquel quickly advised me of best practices around how frequent I should take certain medicines. On her next round to my room, my pain had not subsided, and I had more questions. New questions, as my mind raced.

"I think I need something stronger, but I'm nursing. Is this going to hurt my baby?" I asked. Every time she came back, I thought of something new and wanted to understand what was happening even though no one could say what exactly was wrong with me.

I was there for two days when I thought I might be headed home before a terrible experience in the bathroom where I found myself unable to stand up after using the toilet. My husband called to the nurses for help, they and the support staff came with a wheelchair.

I was helped to the chair and placed on my bed. The slightest movement made me feel like I was being stabbed and my body felt weak and in pain all over as they tried to aid me. I couldn't isolate the feelings to one place like my torso, limbs or even any organs. The slightest movement made me feel like my whole body was gripped by a paralyzing pain. "Don't move!" was the only clear thought I had.

When I finally got in the bed I tried to stay as still as possible. I thanked the staff for their help and tried to articulate what I was feeling so they could assist me.

The nurse rushed me more pain meds but gave me the unfortunate news that I would not be heading home and instead would need to be admitted to the hospital.

I missed my son's 1-week old birthday celebration and wasn't sure when or if I would see him again. *'Why don't they know what's wrong with me?'* I thought. *'Will they figure it out before it's too late?'* The pain felt like what I would think death to be.

My nurse encouraged me to pump so that my breast milk wouldn't dry up, but depression was taking over my thoughts. Raquel knew that I wanted to nurse my son and was trying to keep me on track. I couldn't bear the thought of not going home to my son nor the need to stay in the hospital another night during the holidays.

Despite how terrible the situation was, the experience was made much better thanks to the great care I was receiving from my nurse. The care was tied directly to our ability to communicate freely and contextually.

It wasn't just about being able to communicate my pain but getting to know her personally and feeling like she was a person who knew and cared about me too.

Raquel could hear my fears, she knew what they

were, and she spoke to them. She spoke to me in ways that helped me, about the specific things I needed. At times, she tried to distract me telling me stories that would take my mind off the reality that I was experiencing.

If you have ever been hospitalized then you may be able to relate to my story of having questions and wanting answers, even the simplest ones. Imagine having all those emotions but not being able to communicate with your nurse directly. Many nurses see first-hand the difficulty of care when they can't communicate with their patients in a basic manner.
If you're a nurse, you understand personally the lack of connection or your ability to serve patients that you can't communicate with directly. Something as simple as being able to ask a patient if they need to use the bathroom on your rounds is very useful. Having to get a translator tool like a phone or tablet or find a colleague for something so simple is distracting and slows down your ability to work and get your rounds done.

If you're a hospital administrator, you may know horror stories of avoidable mistakes if only a little more communication was available at a critical moment in care. You may have also heard from staff about technical issues with translator tools and how they can be cold and reduce the quality of a patient's hospital experience.

With Covid-19, the emotions associated with a hospital visit are even more heightened. The pandemic has exacerbated many issues from regular hospital experiences for nurses and patients from emergency rooms to long stay-hospital rooms. Problems that were easier to deal with on a normal scale have become a greater challenge just by sheer volume.

With all these things to consider, not being able to communicate with a patient because of a language barrier could mean life or death in an already delicate situation. It could also mean comfort and peace through a difficult experience which is a pillar of what nurses do in hospitals and with after hospital care already.

About the book
This book is not a plea for nurses to be able to become certified Spanish Interpreters, nor a request for nurses to be able to communicate full medical procedures. It rather makes the case for a basic ability to communicate key phrases to enhance the therapy that nurses provide on a regular basis which aids in recovery and makes more people feel safe coming to the hospital knowing they will be well taken care of.

This book provides a strategy to use a tool (music) to not only learn some basic phrases in Spanish but to keep learning and remember them. Unlike a classroom, this method provides an easy stress-free way to keep developing and remembering Spanish words as you decompress.

This book, "…Learn Spanish with Music for Nurses," was written when hospitals around the US have ICU beds at 97%+ capacity and patients in hallways normally reserved as walkways. The singular goal of the book is to ease the stress for both nurses and their patients when they want to communicate on a basic level.

If you've already tried learning Spanish several times, this book helps you access the Spanish you already know so you can remember it and use it when you need to. As certain as you start dancing when you hear the first few beats of Despacito (even if you've only heard the Justin Bieber version). This book teaches proven strategies to take the Spanish music you love and use it as a tool to communicate with your Spanish-speaking patients.

If you're a nurse or if you know a nurse who could benefit from less stress trying to communicate at work give this book a try! Learn while you relax in a way that really helps you remember Spanish so you can use it when you need it most.

For nurses who need assistance figuring out which songs they like or want premade songs for learning Spanish terminology you can also visit YouTube and search for VocabBlocks or go to VocabBlocks.com for resources and cheat sheets.

Learning Spanish vs. Speaking Spanish

So many people, not just nurses, have "learn Spanish" as something they hope to do before they die. Something they've placed on a proverbial 'bucket list.' The real interest is not just to learn some words and how conjugations work but to be able to speak confidently with natives when you need to communicate something.

If you've tried to learn Spanish before, whether having studied a little or a lot, you know that remembering words and only using them within a learning app, with a Spanish teacher or in a Spanish class is not the same as being able to communicate in Spanish.

You may have been able to remember the words long enough to pass a test or accelerate to the next level in the app but if you cannot remember any of the words when you're ready to communicate it's time to try something new.

Studying without speaking to natives is the reality of where many language lessons stop, even if someone has a great deal of knowledge. You may know someone who has majored or minored in the Spanish language in college but will not use what they know to speak to a native. I know a few of those people myself.

In one instance, the person (my husband, but let's pretend we don't know that) had a minor in Spanish and even taught the language over the summer to middle school students. But with all his knowledge, he makes no attempts to use the language so it's buried in the back of his brain and he doesn't feel like he can really speak Spanish. On a trip to Mexico in 2019 he wouldn't say more than "gracias" to anyone we spoke to.

Meanwhile, I was able to check-in to the resort speaking only Spanish. We were given instructions asked preferences and when the front desk clerk checked in to confirm I understood everything he said in Spanish he was delighted by my abilities. He appreciated it so much that we got a room upgrade. That meant we were closer to all the attractions and received more perks.

My husband isn't the only person I know who *'knows'* Spanish but doesn't feel comfortable *speaking in Spanish*.

In another instance, I was out at brunch with a bunch of friends from business school yapping away in Spanish with the waiter. After we left the restaurant, one of my classmates mentioned that she had majored in Spanish while in college and knew exactly what I was saying. "Really?!" I responded in shock. Why didn't you say anything? Her response was something like "I don't like using it"

After having studied and studied both people lack the confidence to use what they learned. If you're a knower but not a doer this book will help you too!

This book's purpose is to help you move from knowing Spanish to speaking Spanish with confidence and comprehension.

Chapter Two:
Capítulo Dos
Language Short Circuit

Use Your Phone

Have you ever watched the show "90-Day Fiancé" on TLC? The show features couples who are having cross continental relationships. One of the lovers is based in the United States and their future spouse lives in another country. The person based in the United States brings their international lover to the U.S. on a sponsored temporary spousal visa. The visa gives the couple 90-days to get married or the international lover is supposed to return home.

Long-distance dating makes for great Reality Television, but when you add the fact that some couples don't speak the same language you've got a hit in what many would consider unbelievable, must-watch television.

If you've ever tried to have a healthy relationship with anyone, a sibling, parent, friend, lover. You know the important role communication plays in the success of the relationship. Even with the best efforts speaking the same language sometimes wires get crossed and communication falls short.

Imagine the added stress that is placed on a relationship when you need to rely on a phone to speak with your loved one.

90-Day Fiancé has featured multiple couples who don't speak the same language and need help to communicate. They meet online through international dating websites which conveniently translate their conversations. When they meet in person, they opt to use their phones.

The first couple I saw doing this was Paul, a guy from the US, and Karine, a Brazilian woman who he met online. Paul spoke no Portuguese and Karine spoke a little English when they first started dating.

The show filmed their interactions on Paul's first trip to Brazil. A few days after they were face to face Paul wanted to move the relationship to the next level and become intimate. He used his phone to communicate this to Karine in addition to a little concern he had.

Paul spoke in English into his phone, "I want you to be tested for sexually transmitted diseases before we have sex." The app translated his words as he handed his phone to Karine so she could read what he just said. Her face flushed with embarrassment and anger and she immediately responded to his request with disappointed stares and quickly flowing words in Portuguese.

Is this the best way to have this sort of conversation? Does the technology help or create a crutch that stops people from using their brains all together? I know what you're thinking, there's better technology. They should use an app that does more.

Eventually, their communication got an upgrade

when they started using apps that spoke the translations of what they were saying out loud so that their partner no longer needed to read it. But, not surprisingly they continued to find themselves in hostile confrontations.

It's not just what you say but also how you say it that matters. Your tone of voice, your facial expression and the words you use all blend together to communicate the depths of the message you are sharing. Saying anything through a phone limits your ability to be effective.

It's been said that, in life, you are either growing or dying. So that we should constantly be looking for ways to develop our skills instead of ways to be lazier and shut our brains down. Allowing technology to speak for us is not a way of growing.

Crutches

In hospitals, crutches are used to help support someone with a temporary short-coming. They are not meant to replace the person's ability to support themselves for the rest of their lives. When it comes to communication, translator tools can also be a debilitating crutch that stop people from using their brains when working with patients who don't speak the same language as they do.

On one hand, it's an absolute gift to be able to communicate with someone who speaks a language you don't understand with technology. However, there are points in communication where technology is not the best option.

Besides the inability to communicate directly which would be more intimate. Translator tools are notorious for getting things wrong. In theory, being able to look up a vocabulary word or get clarity about something on the spot when trying to speak another language is useful.

Languages often have more than one use for their words. Take the word 'que,' for example, in Spanish. It can mean "what, that, than and more." Similarly, there can be several different translations to a word like 'plate.' Google Translate lists more than 20 options.

Like placo – think silver plated, or plato, like the dish you eat on. If you only rely on translator tools to communicate you probably don't have the slightest idea about the possibilities of misinterpretation or where those error points might be.

Beyond a literal translation error possibility, consider how well technology works when we need it the most. My phone usually stops working or develops a glitch right when I need it to come through for me quickly. Like as soon as I step out of the subway in Manhattan and need walking directions to my destination.

Have you ever experienced an internet outage? Or how about a dead cell phone? What about a natural disaster, even a temporary one, that leaves you without electricity or the internet?

How did you feel when it happened? Was it a simple inconvenience or much more? If you have a dependency to communicate using your phone it might be much more significant. Like with Paul and Karine.

The point is if you've developed a crutch it's time to get strong again. Consider the benefits of being able to speak Spanish on your own. Beyond being able to communicate with patients directly to build rapport and increase their assurances during your interaction. There's also a cool factor that comes with being able to communicate in another language.

Second Language Superpower

People who speak a foreign language have a mysteriousness which feels magical. We wonder, *how do they do that*? Looking at people talking, with foreign words and watching them understand each other, leaves monolinguals feeling left out at minimum.

'What are they saying? How can these people do this? Their brains must be amazing. Advanced. They must operate at a higher level of cognition than monolinguals. How can I develop this expanded mental processing

ability?"

We understand how people with a range of experiences can make better decisions in life. From something as simple as when to cross the street.

There's a fast-moving car approaching – my brain, having lived over 30 years, tells me to wait on the sidewalk until the car passes and not cross until I'm sure they're no others coming. My 2-year old nephew sees the situation differently. His range of knowledge and experience is limited.

He thinks wow, that car is driving quickly in the street, I want to run quickly behind it, with no consideration for the danger of that car hitting him or another one that might be driving behind it.

To me, the smartest people have a broad range of references they can lean on to make decisions. Consider emergency room doctors, when someone walks in needing help, they must know about all the parts of the body in order to make an assessment on what tests to run to understand the best treatment options.

If they just know about how the digestive system functions, they would not be able to accurately figure out how to treat a patient with a shoulder injury.

The knowledge and experience of good doctors leads

them to ask questions to understand further what the real issues might be beyond any obvious symptoms.

The brains of multilinguals are processing the world and everything and everyone they know in a unique way because of their language vocabulary. Learning a new language forces your knowledge base to expand.

This broader perspective creates a greater degree of cultural sensitivity. Learning that "leave me alone" in Spanish has a direct translation of "leave me in peace" makes you aware of contextual differences in the language and culture. You think differently.

The reward you feel from being able to communicate in a foreign language makes the case for why taking the time to study is worth it. Making studying a priority helps you feel the progress in the development of your language skills.

The Best Part

In July of 2012, I went to Mexico City for a week to visit a friend from business school, Fabiola, and her family. We planned to stay with her in-laws for the duration of the trip. This was great because Fabiola's in-laws don't speak English. I would be able to practice and improve my Spanish the entire trip. After studying Spanish off and on for many years, I felt confident that I would be able to communicate with them.

Plus, it was a safe environment, no pressure. No need to say everything perfectly. I was sure they would work with me on any words I got wrong or incorrect conjugations. Much to my dismay, I was not able to understand the majority of what they said and had to rely on Fabiola and her husband to interpret for me.

I could pick out a word here or there. Oh, "cocinando" means cooking, right?

From time to time I could also pick up on some of what was being discussed overall. For the most part, we were not able to communicate directly. After making studying a priority, I met up with Fabiola's in-laws again while they were traveling in New York in 2015.

I went to dinner alone with them and was thrilled with all the progress I made. While riding in a taxi to meet them at their hotel Fabiola's father-in-law called me to check-in. I was nervous when my phone rang but ready for the challenge.

"Bueno" I said, when I answered.

I was able to speak with them over the phone completely understanding them. Speaking on the phone is particularly difficult in a foreign language because there are no visual context clues to pick up on. My heart beat fast with excitement while we spoke, and my pride and smile were through the roof as we talked.

Once I arrived at their hotel near Time Square, we walked to dinner and hung out for a few hours that evening. No translators needed. Knowing that only a few years before I was not able to communicate with them, I felt so happy that I had invested to make learning a priority.

Can you think of a time when you wanted to communicate in Spanish, but you couldn't?

If a year from now, you could set yourself up to never miss an opportunity to communicate in a conversation in Spanish would you take some time to learn more?

Visualize yourself celebrating your own progress a year from now or giving excuses for why you still can't communicate. Which feels better?

There are times when it seems like learning doesn't have a purpose beyond one missed moment. Sometimes it's hard to visualize the missed opportunities as nothing more than superficial experiences like being able to pick up a date.

Consider a deeper opportunity like being the only person who could help someone in need. Especially in a hospital setting.

Wherever you are in your journey learning I have probably been there before, from that initial spark of interest, to missing opportunities and eventually getting started and then being distracted by life and getting started again, and again... My learning journey was a roller coaster of highs and lows, learning and losing (or should I say forgetting). If you are anything like me, despite your intentions to become fluent there was always something that got in the way of your learning journey.

Chapter Three:
Capítulo Tres
My Story

Learning Journey

I've loved foreign languages since I can remember. There is a long list of institutions where I've studied foreign languages. From colleges and universities (Manhattanville College, Middlebury College, New York University) to language schools (Berlitz, CELCUM. Instituto Cervantes), to private lessons (Verbling, Polly Lingual) to self-study apps and CDs (Rosetta Stone, Duolingo).

My first memory of being drawn to foreign languages was when I was still in elementary school. It started in a storage space under my house that us kids decided to play in without permission. I loved playing with the older girls on my block. On this day, they must have wanted a break from my younger nagging ways so they created a secret language to communicate in so that I wouldn't know what they were talking about.

'Fascinating!' I thought. I was mesmerized by not knowing what they were saying, and I wanted to have the same ability to speak in a secret language.

Of all the impressionable experiences of my childhood this one stood out most for me. I wanted to know what they were saying, and what the corresponding English word was for each word I heard. I needed to be able to switch languages myself.

My first chance at learning a new language came shortly thereafter. While participating in an afterschool program one of the teachers offered to teach us sign language. 'Finally!' I thought. 'I join a secret society.'

The day of the first lesson, I showed up with a big smile and eyes wide open as I mimicked the teacher's hand movements. I memorized the entire alphabet in the first week. My desire to be able to speak another language only grew more.

Once I entered middle school, I thought I would finally have the chance to learn to speak a new language. My middle school offered three different foreign languages; Spanish, Italian and French. I contemplated which language I would study; I knew the class sizes were limited so I figured I would do anyone so long as there was room. My heart sank when my teacher told me that all the classes were full, and I would not be able to take any of them. I had to wait until high school to finally start taking Spanish.

My first year of high school, I looked over my schedule searching for the days and time I would get to learn Spanish. I had butterflies in my stomach the first time I walked in my Spanish class.
'This is it; I'm going to become a multilingual,' I thought. My butterflies flew away within a few lessons. I learned a few things, but I needed more. I had no

idea that the following year I would get what I was looking for.

My second year of high school was an upgrade. My new Spanish teacher, Ms. Sebastian, had recently graduated with her master's degree and was back teaching at the school she had graduated from only a few years before. Being so close in age to us students gave her a cool factor that most other teachers didn't have.

My high school, Mount Vernon High School, was a predominately black school but the faculty did not look like the student body. Ms. Sebastian was a unique case in that she did look like us. She was black and Latina, and had lived in the Dominican Republic during college. As a bonus, she spoke Spanish and didn't just teach it.

Ms. Sebastian was committed to making sure we learned well and retained what we were learning. In her class we had to work at our highest capabilities. Ms. Sebastian took our lessons outside of the classroom and had us go to a local Spanish restaurant to practice our speaking ability. We ordered our food speaking Spanish only with the waiters. This was not a required activity, but it was so much fun, and Ms. Sebastian was so loved by her students that just about everyone attended.

I was as dedicated to my learning and my teacher as

she was to us. I skipped a family vacation to stay home and study for a test one weekend thanks to my excitement around finally learning. I built up a great sensibility in the language that year. It gave me a solid foundation of the basics, but I didn't have many opportunities to keep practicing and learning more after that year ended.

When I got to college, I had a unique encounter which can be credited for the concept of this book. A profound learning experience which happened outside of the classroom.

A Latina classmate of mine, Ella, wanted me to braid her hair. I agreed to do it in exchange for her teaching me some Spanish. After some back and forth we decided the best way for me to learn would be if she wrote down the lyrics to a song while we listened to it as I braided her hair. That way she could explain the meaning of the lyrics to me and I could practice singing the song on my own later to learn and remember the Spanish vocabulary.

I gave her some index cards and she played the song while she wrote the words down in Spanish explaining to me all long what was being said. She also gave me some background on the music genre, it was bachata and there was a specific way to dance to it that she showed me as well. I loved the melody and took to the song right away.

As soon as she left my room, I put the song on and started singing along with the lyrics. "It's five in the morning and I haven't slept at all…" I still know all the words to the song Obsession by Aventura to this day.

Since I liked the group so much, I eventually went out and bought one of their albums, "God's Project," on a CD. This was in 2005 – that's what we did back then. I went on to learn the lyrics to additional songs ('Ella y Yo' and 'Un Beso') and continued to build my vocabulary in Spanish.

At the same time, I was navigating through college life, classes, student organizations, part-time jobs, and internships. If you've read my book, *"More than Majors,"* you know that in college I was very ambitious and focused on getting my dream job once I graduated. Learning Spanish was high on my priority list, but it was second to getting my after-college dream job.

I had this great tool, but I hadn't yet realized how valuable it would be to implement it to get me further on my journey towards fluency.

If your story is anything like mine, you probably had something get in the way of your learning journey as well. As you're making your way through life you might start to make excuses for why it isn't worth it to invest the time to learn. This book will help you see how easy it is to learn and make progress developing your ability to speak in Spanish with music.

Street Cred
I found a way to infuse learning into my busy lifestyle. A tool, music, you can use to create an abroad foreign language learning experience for yourself at home. A way to stay consistently engaged in the language effortlessly.

This will help you build vocabulary in a practical and memorable way which helps you remember it when you want to speak in Spanish. This is my super practical approach to move from learning Spanish to using what you know so you don't forget what you've learned.

I am not a certified interpreter, in fact, I'm just a black girl who grew up in a predominantly black neighborhood (where Ebonics was the most commonly spoken language). The high I receive from speaking in Spanish and being understood motivated me to keep learning and now share my learning hacks with you. This book shares what worked for me. I hope you find it useful.

My passion for sharing this information stems from my experiences learning foreign languages, some of which I covered previously, and finally being confident enough in the language to help others. As well as, teaching English. Whenever I hear that someone is trying to learn a new language I think, I can help! With this book I'm hoping to help as many people as possible.

Volunteering

As I confidently transitioned to communicating with native speakers I had more and more rewarding experiences. One of which was, being able to volunteer with an organization, *Languages Without Limits*, that helped individuals and groups who needed interpreters and translators but didn't have budgets for them.

Under that group of volunteers, I had the privilege of volunteering my Spanish skills with schools and organizations that would not otherwise have budgets for Spanish interpreters. In both instances they organizations were making it possible for parents to be more involved with their children's education and care.

Without being connected to Languages without limits the teachers would need to rely on their students to communicate messages to the parents including those around discipline which created a conflict. We also volunteered with an organization that cared for children with disabilities. The organization hosted monthly meetings for the parents but did not have a budget for translation services.

A Different Perspective

As an English teacher I got to explore and understand the complexities of learning a foreign language from the native perspective. As a student I was learning the new words and their rules and had the challenge of sorting through lots of new information. As the teacher I knew all the info and had to help someone else understand it.

Teaching English helped me learn more about language generally and how much we take for granted when we only speak in our native tongue. There are many examples of this, like how many foreign words we've adopted into the English language and all the ways that you can pronounce our words and letters.

Ultimately, teaching English emphasized the need to learn a foreign language with as much of the foreign context as possible. In other words, there are many benefits to learning Spanish from a native Spanish speaker. One point where that strikes home the most for me is with accents.

≠

Some people view the way they speak as a representation of who they are. In turn, when learning a new language, it may be hard for them to truly adapt to the pronunciation of the words because they feel so… well, foreign. For some people it feels like they are impersonating someone else when they speak which doesn't feel good.

Having a native accent sometimes has no effect on understanding but in other instances it can have a big impact.

For instance, one of my native Japanese speaking students went into a store looking to purchase some lip balm. When he roamed the store on his own, he was unable to find it, so he asked a clerk for assistance.

"We don't sell chopsticks." The clerk said to him.

He shook his head 'no' and enunciated slowly ensuring his lips changed shape to help her understand him. "Not, chopsticks, I am looking for CHAPSTICK," he said again.

Was it his pronunciation that through the clerk off or was it an assumption she made in listening? He told me the story during our tutoring session and went on to share more that he noticed.

"Sometimes, I find it hard to understand what people are saying. And it seems they also find it hard to understand me. What I have learned about the English language is not how people speak," he continued. He was right.

At his request, I stopped using my professional speech as much during our sessions and moved to my colloquial way of speaking. Our lessons focused less on the books we were using and took a more conversational approach.

We started talking about our daily lives and I would correct his speech in real time to help him better see some of the mistakes he was making. He, in turn, could stop me when I said something that he didn't understand. Or also mimic my speech to use English that is more commonly spoken than read.

"See there - you said *wanna*. I wanna go to Japan, not *want to*" he would comment.

My case for learning Spanish with music is rooted in the native context. Words spoken in Spanish songs are spoken in the same way that native speakers speak. Many times, they carry a lot of swag and can be more difficult to decipher but they present a more realistic context for learning.

A benefit to moving through language with music in the native context is the ability to put a song on repeat and listen repeatedly. But more on the specific benefits later.

Chapter Four:
Capítulo Cuatro
A Case for Music

The first time I ever learned anything using music was in middle school. It was during my English class, Marty, my teacher was breaking down the meaning of Irony. He used Alanis Morrisette's song, "Ironic," to do it.

This was the most enjoyable day of English Class ever, for me. He started the class by playing the full song. It was a pleasure to listen to, nothing like the learning songs I heard in other classes which I found, at a minimum, corny and boring.

Alanis was not boring - yay! He handed out the lyrics. Gave us a chance to read them and then went back through the song with us line by line.

"Okay, why is this ironic?" he asked. "No, one wants rain or their wedding day" a student called out.

"And what's ironic about this?" he asked about another line of the song "He finally decided to fly, and his worst fear happened," a student responded.

The lesson was engaging and relevant. Not just because the melody was great, but the lyrics spoke to experiences we have. Music and its lyrics generally capture what's happening to all of us in our real lives.

Things like falling in love, and sometimes falling out of love. Or how we hustle to make our dreams happen, have the best careers and how we overcome fears. We love our families, we have hard times, we cope with them. Music captures the passions of life. Learning with music helps us learn in context.

Learning the vocabulary of a song and singing it, helps us keep the meaning of the words and think about them in a fun context. Using popular music has the benefits of tying meaning to memory. I still know the words to Alanis Morrissett's song, Ironic today more than two decades later.

Using music as a tool for learning gives you a way to keep studying and remembering vocabulary in a low-pressure environment. Choosing to listen to a song in Spanish while commuting home after working doesn't make you feel like you're studying after already being exhausted from a long day of work. It's a pleasurable way to get a boost from a melody while contextually placing your brain in an abroad experience.

With all the benefits of knowing how to speak Spanish, why don't more native English Speakers confidently speak in Spanish?

» *Part Two* «

Why does learning a new language allude so many? Why does it seem so impossible? Do you really have to wait until retirement to learn a new language? Is fluency only possible if you move abroad? Let's understand some of the issues that are holding us back so that we can push past them.

Chapter Five:
Capítulo Cinco
Lies We Believe

Kids Can, Adults Can't

"Only Children are truly capable of learning a new language."

Have you heard that one before? Have you been using it as an excuse not to try to learn a new language on your own? I believe this idea is misconstrued. There are benefits to learning a new language as a child but there's no proof that adults cannot learn a new language as well.

Instead of writing off an adult's ability to learn Spanish let's try making a different consideration around how adults and children learn.

What if the way adults and children learn are just different? Compare it to the context of a memoir vs that of a scripted story. Or a scripted television show versus reality tv. Meaning, adults learn in a scripted defined way, like a scripted story. While children learn in a liberal manner like a story from someone's memoir.

I fed into this belief at the tender age of 22. I thought I had missed my opportunity to ever become fluent in Spanish. Until I remembered that my mother changed her life and became a nurse at the age of 39, as a divorced mom of four working two jobs. By the time I turned 28 my Spanish abilities had a major upgrade and I was convinced anyone could learn just like I did at any age.

It's not that adults can't learn another language; we just use different contexts. Process and digest the information differently. So, don't believe the hype. You can learn another language at any age. You just need to make the process of your learning work for you.

No Good at Languages

Or maybe you've heard or said, "I don't have a brain for language learning." This might be a good time to say that if I can do it anyone can do it. Since I didn't score that high or my SATs nor GMAT. But I just stuck with it.

Still, if you're convinced only a certain kind of brain learns languages this one may be harder to get over for you. Consider that when we first learned how to speak in English, we weren't that good at that language either.

Think of a child's mistakes which are corrected by loved ones. There's the super cute stuff that just doesn't connect, like when my son asked if he could sleep in "mybed" when he wanted to sleep with me. He didn't understand that I was saying two words. Or that when speaking about my bed he needed to say your bed. But now that he's three years old, he's somehow figured that part out.

He still makes plenty of mistakes though. I personally continued to make mistakes speaking through elementary school which my parents repeatedly corrected.

We kids would speak among each other before an adult intervened.

"I be running fast before the ball hits me." I might say. Before my dad said, in his most disgusted voice, "I be?" That was enough for me to know I needed to correct that part of the sentence.

Most people are not that good at anything they do when it's new. You can consider the ability to speak in a new language as something people are naturally good at, which would lead you to believe that you simply can't do it because you don't know how or you could consider that anything can be learned with effort. I urge you to focus on the latter.

Effort is the way to learn anything in life and ensure continued improvement. Considering only natural talent robs us of our ability to keep growing, being more and learning more. We can try to learn something new, do something more, become something different than we are today. Effort helps us become the best version of ourselves constantly.

If you want to understand the benefits of focusing on your efforts instead of what anyone deems a natural ability, consider reading Carol Dweck's book "Mindset."

If you've believed the lie about 'just not being good at languages', there may be other limits that you're unnecessarily placing on yourself. Reading Dweck's book might just be the reality check that frees you to grow to the next level of your personal/professional/romantic existence.

Adopting either of these viewpoints on your ability to learn versus a child or your natural abilities are the first hurdle to jump over to get your mind open to what you can achieve.

Once you believe you can learn, your ability to take in the possibility of doing it will flow much more naturally.

Chapter Six:
Capítulo Seis
Inspiration Lost

When you start your language learning journey, you probably never think "I'm going to pay for this class and then let life distract me from actually attending the lessons before the halfway point."

Or, I'm going to buy this Rosetta Stone learning kit, and never even open the box. But somehow, in one way or another we lose the inspiration that was once burning in the beginning inspiring us to learn in the first place.

No Time

There's just not enough time in the day... Sound familiar? Feeling short on time is a great inspiration killer. We feel a struggle between what we need to do and what we want to do.

We quickly assess how much we need the language right now. And the worst idea we might add to that is I'm probably not going to be able to learn enough to use this soon anyway so I might as well focus on something that has a more immediate result.

Language learning often takes a back seat to more immediate needs like working, going to school and spending time with family and friends.

But then you have a Spanish-only speaking patient and you think, I would love to just ask this patient if they're hungry or want something to drink. Just like I've asked all my other patients. But you don't because you don't know how to say it, and while you might use your phone, ironically, you left it at home today.

Looking back on the time that past from when you first started learning you consider how far you could be if you just gave a little more effort to developing your Spanish skills.

Constant Starter

At the beginning of my learning journey I took Spanish 1 so many times, that it didn't make sense. I would often know the information that the teacher was covering but didn't have the confidence to jump into the next level.

I was sure that since so much time had passed since my last class, I needed to start again from the beginning to relearn everything. Everything that I was sure I probably forgot.

If you're like me and If you've given up in the past after being distracted by life and tried again but felt it was impossible to find the time, and then started again with a different system/school/teacher you may feel discouraged by always being a starter.

Don't worry, all your 'starts' will be beneficial with the method of learning with music.

Using this strategy decide in advance that you will

commit this time. As you've seen, you'll only be back soon anyway. I am going to give you many options to make sticking with it as easy as possible.

Lack of Comprehension

Maybe you feel like you gave learning Spanish your best effort and it just feels impossible. "this is too hard," you thought. We've already talked about mindset issues – the belief that you "just can't do it."

If you're not coming from that place and are frustrated by some other issues like how fast Spanish-speakers talk. Or your ability to understand different accents. Know that I hear you! There are tools that can help you get past these issues.

In the moments that matter, when someone is sick and needs help, I'm sure they wouldn't mind you asking them to speak more slowly. Using music to learn Spanish puts you in the thick of accent comprehension.

Another tool is to ask clarifying questions. I find myself using the Spanish I know to confirm that I understood what the person just said to me.

No Progress

Studying and not seeing or feeling like you're not making any progress is a great de-motivator. When you've studied hard then get around natives and feel discouraged because you can't understand them. It can make you feel that there's no point in studying.

Why would anyone want to keep doing anything if they're not seeing results? Maybe we can take a different perspective on this one too.

Compare it to going to college and not being able to get a job after the first year is completed. Would you want to drop out and try something more lucrative like selling drugs?

Or how about going to the gym, running around in a circle then realizing you haven't lost any weight. Depending on who you are, you might go home and never want to go back. But, if you delay your check-in for a month, you might have a completely different result as well as a routine that feels natural and helps improve your health for the long term.

There are benefits to taking that first step in learning if you stick with it, like getting internships. Which not only gives you some experience in trying a new career but also builds up your resume. Fluency might not happen right away but being able to talk at all is a great start. Talking to more people means getting more comfortable and eventually you'll be comfortable asking for anything you need.

Mistakes

There's a silent killer for stunting growth in language learning. It's not using what you've learned for fear of sounding stupid. Advancing in a foreign language comes from using it. Get comfortable making mistakes.

There was a time when you were less hard on yourself about looking silly, when you first learned how to walk. If you were critical of your ability then, or how silly you looked or the fact that you kept falling I'm sure you would still be crawling today.

How do you treat babies you see as they try to walk today? Do you think, *"you've got to get yourself together baby, this falling down is going to ensure you never have a prom date?"* Or do you think, *"how cute"* as they stagger across the room.

Give yourself a break while you're learning and growing in the language. Although people may laugh at you a little it's only because they think the mistake you're making is cute. Well at least that's what you should tell yourself.

Later I'll share some tips for how you can create a safe environment for yourself to make errors so that you don't cheat yourself out of growth.

Context

Learning in a classroom has its benefits, especially when building a foundation of the language. Your classroom experience is even more beneficial if you have a native speaker as your teacher.

On the other hand, classrooms have a way of being lullaby boring. If you can't stay awake for the lesson, there's a high likelihood you won't learn what you need. If the references the teacher uses are completely unrelatable there's a high likelihood you won't remember them. If you're able to learn them at all.

If your classroom is engaging and you can learn, you will be able to develop a better foundation of understanding in the language. Music is a great next step for language development and using what you've learned so you don't forget it.

If your classroom is not as ideal, learning 'textbook Spanish' from a non-native speaker is a recipe for never feeling confident listening to or speaking with native speakers.

Just like with my Japanese student, learning the textbook version of a language can only get you so far. Hearing natives speak with slang and varied word usage is what makes comprehension more true-to-life.

Why

Take a moment now to write somewhere why you want to learn Spanish. Is it because you want to be able to speak with patients? Would there be an additional benefit you would have from knowing it? Consider the ways your life would be different if you learned Spanish.

How would knowing the language benefit you?

Get specific here. What's one specific instance where you wished you knew Spanish? What would have been different that day if you were able to say a few more words? Were you at work needing help so you had to call on a co-worker? Were you trying to help someone or just trying to figure out what someone was talking about?

Excuses Be Gone

Just remember, with enough effort, you can learn anything. Learning with music has many benefits; including, an opportunity to listen to natives and start getting used to accents plus more.

You don't have to take the easy way out with your phone. It could easily become a crutch. You're the growth minded type, willing to stretch and be more instead of being limited. The reality is, you can develop your foreign language skills using music; with low effort and high impact.

When it comes to learning versus time, the method we're about to discuss works with the lowest commitment of time from a busy lifestyle. Using music to develop foreign language skills quickly changes the process of learning into simply living.

Now keep reading, the information in this book will help you develop your strategy to use music to learn Spanish.

» *Part Three* «

Chapter Seven:
Capítulo Siete
Solution Overview

Have you ever heard someone say that they learned to speak English by listening to music? I was watching a reality tv show called The Voice when a contestant (Marina Chello) mentioned that she learned how to speak English from singing Mariah Carey Songs. Here's a bit from the Voice's website on her experience:

"Marina and her family moved to New York from Uzbekistan in search of a better life when she was 11. Adjusting to the new culture was difficult, but listening to American music helped her learn the language and begin to make friends." (https://www.nbc.com/the-voice/credits/credit/season-17/marina-chello)

She's not the only person I've heard say that. Netflix hosted a reality tv show called Love is Blind. Contestants met and got to know each other through a wall. Some people fell in love without ever seeing each other. The show went on to document what happened after they saw each other and had a chance to spend time together.

One of the contestants, Giannina Gibelli, born in Venezuela, mentioned that she too had learned English from listening to music.

Giannina was quoted saying, *"I learned with Christina Aguilera, Britney Spears, like all of those songs were the way I learned how to communicate and learn expressions. But because I was just kind of immersing myself in it, I* was able to just graduate from ESOL in like two to three months. And people were in there for like a year," on cheatsheet.com (https://www.cheatsheet.com/entertainment/love-is-blind-giannina-gibelli-why-family-left-venezuela-our-apartment-would-get-broken-into-all-the-time.html/)

What if you could remember vocabulary from the Spanish language the way you remember the lyrics to a favorite song?

Pop quiz: Do you remember your favorite song from middle school?

Mine was "Killing Me Softly" by the Fugees. I remember being on the school bus coming back from a school game singing, or rather screaming, with my teammates at the top of our lungs, "Whooooooooooaaaaaa ooooh, whooaaaaa whoooaaaah whoaaaaaa wah wah ha ha... la la la la la la whooooo hooooo oh la la la..."

You get it... Music takes you to a place. You remember the way you felt when you heard it. And if you took the time to really learn the lyrics it's hard to forget them.

Maybe you have a song from a different time period that has a strong hold on you. You remember what you were doing, who you were dating or who you had a crush on. Hearing a song might even remind you of a certain fragrance that someone special wore.

Let's harness the power of music as the solution to your language learning block.

Learn with Music

If you really want to learn Spanish, and get comfortable using it to speak with natives, I advocate you try my method of using music to help you. Music as a language learning tool offers many opportunities to advance in the language. Using music, you can develop vocabulary, get used to native speech, sing-along to develop your pronunciation and confidence, among other benefits.

As the saying goes, if you don't use it you lose it. This method will help you find time to develop and practice your Spanish so that you don't forget it despite a busy lifestyle. You can finally stop being a perpetual beginner and make some progress.

Since this learning is happening with music it may be obvious to you that we'll be developing some good listening skills; but this methodology will also develop your speaking, reading, and writing skills in Spanish as well all in a native context. Ultimately, the greatest emphasis will be placed on speaking and listening.

Learning Lifestyle

Whether you're a student, young or seasoned professional, a new mom or dad or a veteran with a growing family, no one ever feels like they have enough time. We're always so busy. Well, too busy to learn a new language anyway.

Learning with Music provides a way to infuse learning into your busy lifestyle; so, you can learn while you live. You don't have to wait until you retire to learn and get good at speaking in Spanish.

No Extra Time Needed

Do you listen to music as a part of your regular life? Maybe while you work out? Or while you unwind from a long day? When do you listen to music? What purpose does it serve for you?

Have you ever heard the song Danza Kuduro? The words to the song are in both Spanish and Portuguese. Are you familiar with the lyrics? Do you love the beat?

I love working out to the song, featuring Don Omar, and singing along. Killing, the proverbial, two birds with one stone. Remembering the Spanish vocabulary words around body parts like hand, waist and head. Not to mention taking my work out to the next level as Don Omar reminds me not to get tired.

Knowing the lyrics to the song creates a no-extra-time needed learning scenario. If you'd prefer something more relaxed, maybe you can sing-along to a slower paced song while you commute home at night. Something like 'Yo no se manana," by Luis Enrique, might just put you in the mood to let go of whatever may have happened that day so that you can relax and look forward to whatever the day may hold tomorrow.

You can visit my YouTube channel and listen to premade versions of both songs with their lyrics in English and Spanish here:

Relaxing and listening to music have the same effect, solving two needs with one action. You're going to drive home or take the train home anyway. Why not listen to the lyrics of a song that will help you improve your Spanish along the way.

Learning with music is a super low pressure but effective means to learn. There are no deadlines or tests, other than ones you create for yourself. Once you've got the lyrics memorized you can keep your learning going all day if you listen to music all day.

The Basics

If you picked up this book because you understand the need to learn Spanish, you've likely already made some attempts at learning the language. Whether that was downloading an app, or taking classes in school, you've likely built some sort of foundation in the language but hit a roadblock on your journey towards fluency.

My method of learning with music assumes some basic understanding of the Spanish language Even if you only barely passed a high school Spanish class. That should be enough to get you going.

From this basic level music can help you skyrocket your vocabulary building, listening and speaking skills.

If you don't already have a foundation and understanding of the language you should get one. I would recommend the basics be developed as a part of a structured class or one on one tutoring.

You can also try a learning app (Duolingo or Polly Lingual) to see how comfortable you are with your understanding of the language and then decide if you're ready to boost your understanding of the language with music.

Benefits of Music

I've given a few examples of the power of music from its ability to keep you in a native context while learning to its ease implementation into your already fully busy schedule. Here I'll break down the examples further.

Life Inspired Lessons

Songs capture real-life scenarios and, in some instances, describe what happened. Music is a form of storytelling placed on a melody, the ability to learn from listening is like learning from a great story.

A great example is a song featuring Don Omar and Aventura called "Ella y Yo." In the story, Don Omar is explaining to Romeo Santana, Aventura's lead singer, that he's in love with a woman but that this love is forbidden.

Don Omar goes through all the details of this love affair and you get to listen in as Romeo gives him advice. Romeo Santana encourages him to fight for the love that he has with this woman even though she's married.

The lyrics from the chorus repeat. So, once you've got them down you can sing-along. Even if you don't learn the words to every single line of the song knowing the lyrics to the chorus helps you stay involved in the story. You could learn and remember the Spanish word(s) for "fight, advice, love, maybe, heart" and more.

As you become engrossed in the story you may find yourself telling Don Omar to fight for this love affair too. That is of course, until you get to the end of the song when you realize that the woman Don Omar is in love with is Romeo Santana's wife. At which point, your jaw may drop in shock and the lyrics become even more memorable for you because of the shock factor.

When you're ready to move on to your next song you'll be able to bring your understanding of these lyrics and learn more as you continue to develop your vocabulary.

Native Context (Teachers vs Speakers)
The first time I listened to "Ella y Yo." I heard words that I'd never learned before in any Spanish class. Slang words, which had double meanings.

In my opinion, it's beneficial to listen to any genre of music you like to learn Spanish. I don't think it should exclusively be songs where only "proper" Spanish is spoken. Unless you're learning as a diplomat and want to use the words you learn in connection to some high office.

Ideally, I would suggest listening to artists from the country you intend to communicate with most. So, for example, if you're learning Spanish to be able to communicate with the patients in your hospital and they are majority from Venezuela, listening to artists from Venezuela would prove the most valuable.

If you have lots of friends from the Dominican Republic that you'd like to communicate with, it might be better to learn to speak Spanish from a

Dominican artist. This will help you start getting used to their accents, phrases, slang and key words.

≠

I told a Spaniard friend of mine, Alejandro, that I was writing this book and he immediately freaked out at the idea of me teaching people Spanish with Reggaeton.

"That's not real Spanish" he reminded me.

Alejandro and I met while I was living in London. He constantly reminded me that my English was no good too since I'm from New York. I needed to learn to speak the Queen's English.

Whenever I spoke in Spanish with Alejandro, he lovingly tried to get me to develop a lisp. I'm half joking.

Many Spanish words spoken by Spaniards sound like they are speaking with a lisp. The history of this has something to do with a king they once had who spoke with a lisp. To honor his highness, the people mimicked his speech. That's the story I heard. It seemed to make sense to me, but I have zero desire to fact-check that.

I accept the simple truth that if you want to speak with Spaniards to learn from a Spaniard. Otherwise, you might be distracted by the way they are speaking which would only make comprehension more difficult.

My highest comprehension in Spanish is with Mexicans. Many of my Spanish teachers were Mexicans. I understand their accents and slang best. I've even had full on lessons about why the words Madre (mother in Spanish) and Padre (father in Spanish) are used so often in their slang.

Learn and Remember

When I hear a new song that I like I will play it over and over on repeat. There are many factors that pull me in. It can be as simple as relating to the situation being discussed. Or the song could be inspirational with motivation to strive towards my dreams.

When the song is in Spanish, and I've learned the lyrics, I can sing along on every spin. This drills the vocabulary into my brain without even trying. So that once I've learned the vocabulary, I keep remembering them and keeping the language at the front of my brain.

It's an ultimate guide to use it so you don't lose it.

A classic Spanish song I love is Celia Cruz's "Life is a Carnival." It helps me remember that bad times pass. I also learned a lot of vocabulary that repeats in the song. My first time learning the phrase "no hay que" was with this song. That phrase repeats more than a dozen times.

If I'm feeling bad and listen to this song, I find myself encouraged and proud since I'm doing something that I love. Using my Spanish vocabulary. I can confront my situation head on and remember that if I can learn Spanish, I can do anything. You can harness this power too!

If you like to listen to a great song repeatedly this method is going to work well for you.

Fun Education
Have you ever sat in a classroom learning about something and found yourself falling asleep? What about at a conference? Where you needed to get up and get a cup of coffee or just walk for a bit so that you didn't start snoring?

A language lesson based in a song from a genre you like has an extremely low likelihood of putting you to sleep. Unless you intend for it to. Like some smooth music to help your brain think in Spanish as you go to sleep.

When you think of studying in the traditional context do you have the same feelings as when your favorite song starts playing? What if the idea of studying Spanish felt as good to you as going out dancing with friends? It can.

Once you've got the lyrics down, this is the most effortless learning you can do with a fringe benefit of really remembering what you've learned after.

Chapter Eight:
Capítulo Ocho
Formula Breakdown

Vocab as Building Blocks to Convos
More Vocabulary = More Communication

The formula covers four areas of learning: listening, speaking, reading and writing. The greatest emphasis will be placed on both listening and speaking to help you build confidence and be ready to comfortably speak to natives in Spanish.

This formula also focuses on building vocabulary. Having a range of vocabulary to draw from has helped me personally communicate better with anyone comfortably.

While speaking with a native, if I'm unable to understand what they are saying, I can ask clarifying questions to figure out what the conversation is about.

Lack of comprehension for me may be because they are using a word or phrase I don't know, or their accent isn't familiar to me.

Once I clarify what was being said, I often have a new opportunity to develop my language ability by adopting the new word or phrase.

This question asking also can lead to opportunities to supplement in vocabulary to understand what someone is saying. More vocabulary = more opportunities to communicate. More on this next.

Es Como = It's like
Here's one example of how I use the words I know to describe what I need if I don't know how to say it.

Let's pretend that you don't know the word for 'ice' in Spanish, but your drink is warm, and you'd like to ask for some. Here are two ways you might be able to use vocabulary you know to ask for ice.

You might say "my drink is not cold" or "my drink is warm" and get a response "would you like some ice?" In case that's not the response you receive, you could try something else. "I don't know the word for it, but I'd like something cold to put into my drink"

The more vocabulary you have the more you can explain or describe what you're trying to say while communicating with a native Spanish speaker. Developing vocabulary gives you more pieces of the language puzzle to put together to increase your ability to communicate.

Here's a breakdown of the formula which works if you have a general grasp of the language:
1. Find songs/artist that you like
2. Google the lyrics to the songs
3. Read along to compare the accuracy of what you've found
4. Translate the lyrics
5. Sing-along with the lyrics
6. Memorize the lyrics

Let's get into each step in more detail.

Step One: Artists, Songs & Genres

1. **Identify an artist or songs in a genre you like.**

There is a list of songs and artists in the appendix at the back of this book. That's a great place to start if you haven't already identified some favorites. The list is also available for download on my website if you'd like to share with a friend who really needs some help getting their Spanish upgraded. If for some reason, you're unable to find a song or artist you like email me ing@ingersinfo.com and I'll help you find some.

Select one song to focus on initially. Ideally, this is a song that you would like to listen to repeatedly without growing tired of it. Having some basic understanding of the language it's likely there will be several words you can recognize that first go around even if you don't remember the meaning of the words.

Take a full listen to the song and see what words, if any, you can recognize as familiar. Before moving on to step two, write down all the words you can identify and their meanings on the first go around to see if you can understand what is being said. This will begin the process of independently sharpening your listening skills.

Step Two: Lyrics

2. Find the lyrics.

This is the first step in vocabulary development via learning with music. Researching vocabulary. Here you start to get familiar with the new Spanish words.

When searching for the lyrics, type the name of the song into a search engine (I usually use Google) and at the word "letra" which means 'lyric' in Spanish.

While understanding the lyrics for the full song is beneficial. It may be best to focus on the lyrics to the chorus initially before trying to understand or memorize the entire song.

That said, feel free to have a look at the full lyrics to the song initially. You know your grasp of the language, don't overwhelm yourself. Doing a little at a time can help you see great progress and keep you motivated to learn more.

The chorus of the song is usually repeated a few times in between versus so learning the chorus provides a double, triple, or quadruple win depending on how many times it is repeated in the given song.

If you're a little intimidated about doing this, start with a slower paced song. If you like R&B music try the 'Dime Remix' featuring Pitbull. You could also try a faster paced song with simple lyrics like 'Danza Kuduro.' The chorus uses vocabulary you've probably heard from any Spanish level one course you've taken and is great for nurses.

As you advance in your language comprehension you should be learning the entire song and singing along. As your language develops you may be able to skip the "translate" step entirely because you know so many words that you don't need to look up their meanings.

Accent Challenge
As this exercise sharpens your listening skills, it will also force you to adjust to different accents. Be deliberate about the songs you listen to.

Research the artist you like and be familiar with their backgrounds. Which country are they from? Are there unique attributes to the way they speak Spanish? Is there anyone you can speak with to learn more about this type of Spanish? It's origins, or the culture of the artist that you like?

Accents contribute to understanding. Think about two different people, one with a heavy accent and one with a light one. Who do you generally understand better? Consider your own accent.

I've always felt like my Latina friends had double

personalities. The one they used when they spoke to me in English and the persona they put on when they spoke Spanish. To me the back and forth was fascinating. Feel free to dig deep and find your inner Latina while you speak in Spanish too.

Remember, learning with music is 'life inspired learning,' that includes the native context with real speech, real accents and rhythms of speech. Mimicking the artist's pronunciation is a good thing here to sharpen your own pronunciation.

Step Three: Accuracy

3. **Compare for accuracy.**
Lyrics found online do not always match the lyrics you hear in a song. Some websites put on lyrics based on their best bet of what they think they hear. Once you've found some lyrics online, listen to the song while reading the lyrics to see if they seem to match to you.

This is a great exercise to sharpen your listening ability with natives. Even if you don't yet know what the words mean you should be able to distinguish if something sounds right. Or if it sounds nothing like what you're reading.

If what you hear doesn't match what you read it might not be a problem. In the next step you'll translate the lyrics so that you at least know what the person who wrote the lyrics thinks is being said.

There can be multiple meanings to words with one sound. In Spanish, the word "que" has multiple meanings including 'what' or 'that,' for example. In English, consider the letter C, and the words see and sea. All sound the same but mean very different things.

Having slightly wrong song lyrics is not a big deal. Knowing the meaning of the words your saying is of the most importance. Singing "tengo un gato en mis pantalones" and knowing that the sentence translates into "I have a cat in my pants" still helps you remember those vocabulary words. Even if the musical artist is singing "My legs dance in my pants," which would be a completely wrong translation.

If your lyrics match your translations, you will be learning and remembering vocabulary to a great beat.

Step Four: Translate

4. **Translate the lyrics**

A simple way to translate the lyrics you find would be by cutting and pasting them into Google Translate. Read the lyrics in English and see if they make sense to you.

If the words are off, remember my note from above on how words may be written incorrectly. Open a new Google Translate page and play around with the words to see if you can find another word that makes the sentence make sense. Trying using some English words that you think should fit and find the Spanish translations to those words.

If the lyrics don't make sense to you that might be the song's intention.

There's a line in Beyoncé's song 'Black Parade" where she says "bees is known to bite" instead of "bees are known to bite" The grammar isn't exactly accurate, but if you were to translate that you could decide to correct it or remain vigilantly aware of the discrepancy while speaking with natives.

Popular music also has a reputation for being filled with landmines of curse words and double uses of language that are foul. If you swear as a regular part of your life this may not be as big of a concern for you, but it's at least good to know when you're doing it.

Once you've got your lyrics down check in with a tutor or native speaking friend to confirm you won't offend anyone using your new words.

If you're a beginner with Spanish or not confident in your ability to do this step on your you can get started today using my try my premade YouTube videos, which are also available on my website at VocabBlocks.com.

Step Five: Mimic

5. Sing along, imitating as much as possible.
Singing along to the song gives you a chance to develop your speech and pronunciation. You can sing in private at home, in the shower – if you're like me. Or maybe while you drive to work or out shopping.

Practicing in private helps you build your confidence saying the words to no one in particular. The more you say them, the more confident you will feel speaking the new language. Try to mimic the artist's pronunciation exactly.

The singing should be fun, so make sure that you're enjoying it. The more you sing the more you'll be prepared to do the next step.

Step Six: Remember

6. Memorize the lyrics.
As you sing along with the lyrics the memorization should come naturally. If you keep saying something, you'll remember it. So, keep the songs you like on repeat. While you drive or ride the bus or train. When you work out and when you're strolling

for groceries or new clothes. This should be the easiest part. Since all you do, at this point, is turn on a Spanish song that you like.

» *Part Four* «

Chapter Nine:
Capítulo Nueve
The *Doing* Challenge

Pop Quiz: Do you think it's better to *know* how to do something well and not do it? Or, is it better to have a general idea of how to do something and start practicing?

I'm advocating for the latter, the more you practice this system the more your language will develop. Now that you've learned about this process don't stop at knowing. Let's get to some doing.

At the beginning of this book I shared stories of individuals who had great knowledge of the Spanish language but were not practicing what they knew. Practicing singing in private should build your courage and confidence.

Use It; Don't Lose It

Once you've memorized the words and you feel comfortable singing along with songs with comfort. It's time to find someone to practice with. Maybe you have native Spanish speaking friends that you can test the waters with. At the beginning it's helpful if you can use Spanglish (speaking both Spanish and English) with one person until you've established a pretty good vocabulary base.

Use the words you have and the knowledge you've developed to start communicating as best as you can. Keep remembering that your best will get better with time.

Correction: Study Buddy

I shared a story at the beginning of the book about how my parents continued to correct my English throughout elementary school. Find a study buddy that you can completely drop your guard around and ask them to correct you when you make mistakes while speaking.

There are people who have spoken a foreign language fluently for years always making the same mistakes because they haven't requested or given anyone permission to help them improve. Don't make that mistake.

Find someone that you can make an agreement with to correct you when you make mistakes. A native speaker who will constantly tell you when your verb usage or tense is wrong.

You can also try hiring a one on one tutor with Polly Lingual (https://pollylingu.al/) or Verbling (https://www.verbling.com/). I recommend those two sites because I've used them myself.

Practice Groups

Find opportunities to practice your language with natives. I like using meetup.com to find groups to practice with. I live in New York and there are large groups that meet up to do language exchanges. If you're in a smaller city be cautious.

Make sure the group is legit and that there are lots of people attending when possible. Make sure the meetups are in public places with lots of traffic and bring friends if you can to ensure your safety.

More than Words

Nurses by trade are great. I know that first-hand because both my mother and sister are nurses. Nurses are always growing and evolving; learning new technology and how to treat new diseases and figuring out better ways to care for their patients.

"Helping people" is a core part of what nurses do. Learning to communicate in Spanish provides even more opportunities for nurses to be their best selves and be able to advocate for and take care of their patients.

If anyone can learn a new language, it's you. You're a nurse. You passed state boards knowing all about medicine and how to make people feel better with and beyond.

Learning enough Spanish to be able to communicate with patients and learn about their day is totally possible for you.

» *Appendix* «

Need help finding Spanish songs you like? Try these:

Category	Artist
Bachata	Aventura
Bachata	Monchy
Bachata	Prince Royce
Bachata	Romeo Santos
Bachata	Usher & Romeo
Balada	Alejandro Fernandez ft. Christina Aguilera
Balada	Alejandro Sanz
Balada	Camila
Balada	Gianmarco
Balada	Jesse y Joy
Balada	Río Roma
Balada	Thalia
Cumbia / Ska	Vicentico
Electropop	Enrique Iglesias
Funk	El gran silencio
Funk	El gran silencio
Funk	Los amigos invecibles
Funk	Los amigos invecibles
Gospel	Christine D'Clario
Gospel	Marcos Witt
Gospel	Paul Wilbur
Grupera	Ana Bárbara
Huayno	Gloria Estefan
Jazz	Bebo Valdes y Diego El Cigala

Jazz	Cesária Evora
Jazz	Marc Anthony
Jazz	Paté de Fuá y Natalia Lafourcade
Mariachi	Vicente Fernández
Merengue	Bacilos
Merengue	Chino y Nacho
Pop	Bacilos
Pop	Belanova
Pop	Camila
Pop	Carlos Baute ft. Marta Sanchez
Pop	Casi Ángeles
Pop	Diego Torres
Pop	Don Omar y Lucenzo
Pop	Enrique & amigos
Pop	Fanny Lu
Pop	Ha-Ash
Pop	Juanes y Nelly Furtado
Pop	La Quinta Estación
Pop	Marc Anthony
Pop	Natalia y la Forquetina
Pop	Nina Sky et al
Pop	Paulina Rubio
Pop	Plan B
Pop	Reik
Pop	Selena Gomez & The Scene
Pop	Shakira ft. El Cata
Pop	Gloria Estefan
Pop	Laura Pausini
Pop	Omega
R&B	Marc Anthony

R&B	*Omega*
R&B	*Plan B*
R&B	*Prince Royce*
R&B	*Rakim Y Ken Y ft Pitbull*
R&B	*Usher & Romeo*
R&B Latina	*Aventura*
R&B Latina	*Marc Anthony & La India*
R&B Latina	*Omega*
Rap	*Calle 13*
Reggaeton	*Angel y Khriz*
Reggaeton	*Cali y El Dandee*
Reggaeton	*Daddy Yankee*
Reggaeton	*Daddy Yankee*
Reggaeton	*Daddy Yankee*
Reggaeton	*Daddy Yankee*
Reggaeton	*Daddy Yankee ft Wisin Y Yandel*
Reggaeton	*Don Omar*
Reggaeton	*Don Omar y Aventura*
Reggaeton	*Don Omar y MVP*
Reggaeton	*J. Balvin*
Reggaeton	*La Factoría y Eddy Lover*
Reggaeton	*Nicky Jam*
Reggaeton	*Nina Sky et al*
Reggaeton	*Rakim Y Ken Y*
Reggaeton	*Wisin & Yandel*
Reggaeton	*Wisin & Yandel*
Reggaeton	*Gente de Zona & Marc Anthony*
Rock	*Amén*
Rock	*Camila*
Rock	*Enanitos Verdes*

Rock	Héroes del silencio
Rock	Laura Pausini
Rock	Líbido
Rock	Moderatto y Belinda
Rock	Siddhartha
Rock	Soda Stereo
Rock	Soda Stereo
Rock	Zoé
Rock	Zoé
Salsa	Celia Cruz
Salsa	Gente de Zona & Marc Anthony
Salsa	Joe Arroyo
Salsa	La India (aka India)
Salsa	Luis Enrique
Salsa	Marc Anthony
Salsa	Omega
Salsa	Oscar de León
Salsa	Willie Colon y Hector Lavoe
Techno pop	Miranda!
Tropical	Gloria Estefan
Tropipop	Fonseca
Vallenato	Carlos Vives

Below is a list of categories and songs:

Category	Song Title
Bachata	Un Beso
Bachata	Hoja en blanco
Bachata	Darte un beso
Bachata	Propuesta Indecente
Bachata	Promise
Balada	Hoy tengo ganas de ti
Balada	Amiga mía
Balada	Mientes
Balada	Hasta que vuelvas conmigo
Balada	La de la mala suerte
Balada	Me cambiaste la vida
Balada	No me enseñaste
Cumbia / Ska	Los caminos de la vida
Electropop	De noche y de día
Funk	Dormir Soñando
Funk	Chúntaro Style
Funk	Mentiras
Funk	Cuchi Cuchi
Gospel	Padre Nuestro
Gospel	Gracias
Gospel	Conmigo Danza
Grupera	Bandido
Huayno	Hoy
Jazz	Veite Años
Jazz	Bésame mucho
Jazz	Tu amor me hace bien
Jazz	Mi corazón

Mariachi	Me voy a quitar de en medio
Merengue	Mi primer millón
Merengue	Mi niña bonita
Pop	Mi primer millón
Pop	Rosa Pastel
Pop	Perdón
Pop	Colgando en tus manos
Pop	A ver si pueden
Pop	Color Esperanza
Pop	Danza kuduro
Pop	Bailando
Pop	No te pido flores
Pop	Estés donde estés
Pop	Fotografía
Pop	El sol no regresa
Pop	Tu amor me hace bien
Pop	En el 2000
Pop	Oye mi canto
Pop	Mi nuevo vicio
Pop	Si No Le Contesto
Pop	Inolvidable
Pop	Un año sin lluvia
Pop	Loca
Pop	Hoy
Pop	Primavera anticipada
Pop	Estoy Enamorado
R&B	Tu amor me hace bien
R&B	Estoy Enamorado
R&B	Si No Le Contesto
R&B	Stand by my

R&B	Dime remix
R&B	Promise
R&B Latina	Obsesión
R&B Latina	Vivir Lo Nuestro
R&B Latina	Tu no Ta Pa Mi
Rap	Atrévete-te-te
Reggaeton	Ven bailalo
Reggaeton	Yo te esperaré
Reggaeton	Gasolina
Reggaeton	Lo que paso paso
Reggaeton	Rompe
Reggaeton	La Despedida
Reggaeton	Limbo (Remix)
Reggaeton	Dile
Reggaeton	Ella y yo
Reggaeton	Dale don dale
Reggaeton	Ginza
Reggaeton	Perdóname
Reggaeton	Travesuras
Reggaeton	Oye mi canto
Reggaeton	Me matas
Reggaeton	Estoy Enamorado
Reggaeton	Algo me gusta de ti
Reggaeton	La gozadera
Rock	Decir Adiós
Rock	Perdón
Rock	Lamento Boliviano
Rock	La chispa adecuada
Rock	Primavera anticipada
Rock	En esta habitación

Rock	Muriendo lento
Rock	Náufrago
Rock	Persiana Americana
Rock	De música ligera
Rock	Luna
Rock	Soñé
Salsa	La vida es un carnaval
Salsa	La gozadera
Salsa	No le pegue a la negra
Salsa	Mi Mayor Vengaza
Salsa	Yo no se mañana
Salsa	Vivir mi vida
Salsa	Tu Si Quieres, Tu no Quieres
Salsa	Llorarás
Salsa	El día de mi suerte
Techno pop	Perfecta
Tropical	Mi tierra
Tropipop	Arroyito
Vallenato	La gota fría

But wait, there's more…

Get Pre-made videos with lyrics on YouTube: search for "VocabBlocks"

THANK YOU!
PLEASE REVIEW THIS BOOK!

Thank you for taking the time to read this book! It would mean a lot to me if you could leave a review for this book on Amazon!

Your words could help someone else make a decision about getting a copy for their favorite nurse.

www.ingramcontent.com/pod-product-compliance
Lightning Source LLC
Chambersburg PA
CBHW020442220526
45464CB00002B/812